VOCAL EXER
BREATHWORK AN_ ~~~~~~~
TWISTERS

RICHARD CAASI

Copyright © 2023

Table of Contents

Introduction

"The voice is a muscle and needs to be exercised like any other. Warm-ups and vocal exercises are essential for a healthy voice." - Seth Riggs

Welcome to the world of vocal exercises, breathwork and tongue twisters! This book will provide you with the knowledge, guidance, and resources to help you become a better singer or speaker.

Vocal exercises are a great way to improve your singing and speaking ability. They can help you develop your vocal range, improve your vocal power, and increase your confidence. Breathwork can help you manage your breathing and ensure you have the proper technique for singing and speaking. Lastly, tongue twisters are a fun way to practice pronunciation and articulation.

Throughout this book, we will cover the basics of vocal exercises, breathwork, and tongue twisters, and then provide more advanced techniques and tips. We will also provide some fun and creative ways to practice your skills. Whether you are an aspiring or a seasoned professional singer, a teacher, a public speaker or just someone who loves to verbally communicate, this book will help you take your voice to the next level. So let's get started!

Vocal Exercises

Q: What do singers do when they want to warm up their voices?

A: They practice their scales!

What are vocal exercises?

Vocal exercises are exercises designed to strengthen the vocal muscles and improve vocal quality. They can include breathing exercises, lip rolls, tongue twisters, humming, singing scales, and more.

Vocal exercises are an important part of any singer‚Äôs vocal training. They help to strengthen the vocal cords, improve diction and pronunciation, and increase range and resonance. Vocal exercises can also help singers to relax their throat muscles and improve breath control.

The most important thing to remember when doing vocal exercises is to keep your vocal cords in good shape. Start by warming up your voice with some easy scales and then gradually increase the complexity. Use a piano or other musical instrument to help you with the notes. When singing, always use a light and gentle tone, and maintain good posture with your chin up and your shoulders back.

One of the most basic vocal exercises is the lip trill. This exercise helps to develop your breath control and vocal range. Start by taking a deep breath and then slowly make a buzzing sound with your lips. Make sure to inhale and exhale slowly and evenly. You can also use this exercise to practice your diction and pronunciation.

Another vocal exercise is the tongue twister. Start by saying a short phrase or sentence quickly and clearly. Then, try to repeat the phrase three times as quickly as you can, making sure to pronounce each word correctly. This exercise helps to improve your pronunciation and articulation.

Finally, practice the siren exercise. Start with a low note and then gradually increase the pitch until you reach a high note. Make sure to use a consistent and even tone throughout the exercise. This exercise helps to strengthen your vocal cords and improve your vocal range.

Vocal exercises help to improve diction and pronunciation, increase range and resonance, and strengthen the vocal cords. By taking the time to practice these exercises regularly, singers can improve their vocal technique and performance.

Vocal exercises are a great way to strengthen the muscles of the face, throat, and chest, as well as improve vocal range, breath control, and tone. Here are some exercises you can do to get started:

1. Lip Rolls: Start by making a ‚Äúmmmm‚Äù sound, then roll your lips in and out as you make the sound. Concentrate on engaging your lip muscles and keeping the sound even. Do this for 30 seconds, then rest for 30 seconds.

2. Tongue Trills: Make a ‚Äúrrrrrr‚Äù sound with your tongue against the roof of your mouth. Focus on keeping your tongue relaxed

and your sound even. Do this for 30 seconds, then rest for 30 seconds.

3. Jaw Drops: Open your mouth as wide as you can and drop your jaw down as you make a ‚Äúaaaaaah‚Äù sound. Concentrate on keeping your jaw relaxed and your sound even. Do this for 30 seconds, then rest for 30 seconds.

4. Sirens: Start by making a low ‚Äúooooooh‚Äù sound, then gradually increase the pitch of your voice until you reach a high ‚Äúaaaaaah‚Äù sound. Focus on keeping the sound even and consistent as you move up and down the scale. Do this for 30 seconds, then rest for 30 seconds.

5. Yawn-Sighs: Start with a deep breath in, then open your mouth and make a yawning ‚Äúaaaaaah‚Äù sound as you exhale. Focus on keeping your breath even and your sound consistent. Do this for 30 seconds, then rest for 30 seconds.

6. Aum: Start by making the "ahhhh" sound, move into the "ohhhh" sound and finally end with the "mmmmm" sound. There is no pause between the three sounds and each sound should be equal lengths to each other. Hold this sound continuously for as long as you can.

These exercises should be done daily for best results. Be sure to warm up your voice before doing any vocal exercises to prevent strain and injury.

Benefits of vocal exercises

1. Improved vocal range, tone, and resonance.

2. Increased vocal stamina and strength.

3. Improved breath control and airflow.

4. Improved clarity of diction and articulation.

5. Improved vocal projection.

6. Improved intonation and pitch accuracy.

7. Reduced risk of vocal injury.

8. Increased vocal confidence.

A Younger Voice

There are a few techniques you can try to make your voice sound younger:

Practice speaking with more energy and enthusiasm. Younger people often speak with more energy and enthusiasm, so try to infuse your voice with more energy and excitement. Speak with more inflection and enthusiasm in your tone, and try to make your voice sound brighter and more cheerful.

Relax your throat muscles. Younger people often have more relaxed throat muscles, which can create a more youthful sounding voice. Try to loosen up your throat muscles by gently massaging your neck and shoulders, and practice deep breathing exercises to help relax your throat muscles.

Practice speaking in a higher pitch. Younger voices tend to have a higher pitch than older voices, so try to speak with a slightly higher pitch. You don't want to sound like you're speaking in a fake or forced voice, so practice speaking in a higher pitch in a natural way.

Work on your breathing. Younger voices tend to be more breathy and airy, so try to work on your breathing technique to create a more youthful sounding voice. Practice taking deep breaths and exhaling slowly, and try to speak with more airiness and breathiness in your tone.

Stay hydrated. Keeping your vocal cords hydrated can help create a more youthful sounding voice. Drink plenty of water throughout the day, and avoid alcohol and caffeine, which can dehydrate your vocal cords.

Remember that everyone's voice is unique, and trying to sound younger may not necessarily be the best approach for your voice. It's important to practice good vocal hygiene and speak in a way that feels comfortable and natural to you.

Breathwork

"Breathwork is like a bridge between the conscious and unconscious, between body and mind, between action and stillness." - Richard P. Brown, MD

Breathwork is an important component of working with the voice. It is the foundation of proper vocal technique and helps to ensure that the voice is used in a healthy and efficient manner. Breathwork helps to provide the necessary control and power needed to produce the desired sound. It also helps to increase breath capacity and control, which can improve vocal range and tone.

Breathwork is a holistic practice that utilizes the power of breath to promote physical, mental, and spiritual wellbeing. It involves a variety of techniques that use conscious breathing to access and regulate the mind-body connection. Breathwork can be used to reduce stress, help with anxiety, promote healing, and increase self-awareness.

The practice of breathwork has its roots in various ancient spiritual and healing traditions, including yoga and pranayama. It was developed in the mid-20th century by Dr. Stanislav Grof, a psychiatrist and psychotherapist who was one of the pioneers of transpersonal psychology. He believed that conscious breathing could help individuals access and alter their innermost consciousness, providing access to deeper levels of healing and understanding.

In breathwork, practitioners use different types of breathing techniques to access different states of consciousness. These techniques range from rapid breathing to slow, deep breathing and can be used to access different states of relaxation and awareness.

Breathwork has a wide range of potential benefits for people of all ages and backgrounds. It has been found to be effective in treating depression, anxiety, and stress-related issues. It can also be used to increase energy and focus, promote physical healing, and foster emotional and spiritual growth.

Breathwork is a powerful self-care tool that can be used to help people access their own inner wisdom and unlock their potential. It is a safe and gentle practice that can be used by anyone and is available in many forms. From group classes to individual sessions, there are many ways to experience the benefits of breathwork.

Breathwork Exercises

1. Abdominal Breathing

This breathwork exercise is designed to help you relax, reduce stress, and increase your lung capacity. Start by sitting or lying in a comfortable position. Place one hand on your chest and the other on your abdomen. As you inhale, focus on breathing deeply and slowly into your abdomen, allowing your hand to rise. Make sure not to take shallow breaths that only fill your chest. As you exhale, your abdomen should move inward as you release the breath. Continue this breathing pattern for at least five minutes.

2. Ujjayi Breath

Ujjayi breath is a type of breathing exercise used in yoga and meditation. Start by sitting or lying in a comfortable position. Close your eyes and take a few deep breaths. On your next inhale, draw your breath in through your nose and constrict the back of your throat. As you exhale, open your mouth and make an ‚Äúahh‚Äù sound. Repeat this breathing pattern for at least five minutes.

3. Alternate Nostril Breathing

This exercise is designed to help you reduce stress and bring balance to your body. Start by sitting in a comfortable position. Place your right thumb over your right nostril and your ring finger over your left nostril. Close your eyes and take a few deep breaths. Then, inhale through your right nostril and exhale through your left. Repeat this pattern for at least five minutes.

4. Humming Bee Breath

This exercise is designed to help you reduce stress and increase energy levels. Start by sitting in a comfortable position. Close your eyes and take a few deep breaths. Then, inhale deeply and exhale while making a humming bee sound. Make sure to keep your lips closed as you exhale. Continue this breathing pattern for at least five minutes.

5. Bumblebee Breath

This breathing exercise is designed to help you relax and reduce stress. Start by sitting in a comfortable position. Close your eyes and take a few deep breaths. On your next inhale, draw in a deep breath and then exhale while making a bumblebee sound. Make sure to keep your lips closed as you exhale. Repeat this pattern for at least five minutes.

6. Belly Breath

This exercise requires you to stand with your feet hip-width apart and your hands resting on your belly. Take a slow, deep inhalation through your nose and focus on feeling your belly expand as you inhale. Exhale slowly through your mouth and focus on feeling your belly contract as you exhale. Repeat this several times.

7. Singing Breath

Start by standing up with your feet hip-width apart and your arms at your sides. Take a slow, deep inhalation through your nose and as you exhale, sing a scale of your choice. An example would be "Do Re Mi Fa So La Ti Do" where each syllable is a note higher than the previous one. Focus on keeping your jaw relaxed and your lips slightly parted. Repeat this several times.

8. Box Breathing

Box breathing (also known as square breathing or four-square breathing) is a breathing exercise used to reduce stress and anxiety. It involves inhaling for four counts, holding for four counts, exhaling for four counts, and then holding for four counts. This exercise is meant to help focus the mind on the breath and clear the mind of other thoughts. The practice of box breathing can also help slow down an overactive heart rate and relax the body. It is generally recommended that you practice box breathing for at least five minutes a day. If you are feeling particularly stressed, it can be beneficial to practice box breathing for longer periods of time.

Benefits of Breathwork

1. Stress Relief

Breathwork helps to reduce stress, anxiety, and depression by calming the nervous system and allowing you to focus on the present moment.

2. Increased Mindfulness

Breathwork can help you become more mindful and aware of your body, feelings, and thoughts.

3. Improved Physical Health

Breathwork can improve physical health by increasing oxygen intake and promoting relaxation. This can help to reduce pain, improve energy levels, and boost immunity.

4. Emotional Balance

Breathwork can help to regulate emotions, which can be helpful for those struggling with depression or anxiety.

5. Spiritual Connection

Breathwork can help to create a deeper connection to spirit and the divine, as well as a greater sense of peace and connection to the universe.

Tongue Twisters

"Tongue twisters are a great way to sharpen your communication skills and improve your pronunciation." - Unknown

Tongue twisters are fun to say and can be a great way to practice pronunciation. They are also a great way to bond with friends or family over an amusing challenge. A tongue twister is a phrase or sentence that is difficult to articulate because of a succession of similar consonant sounds. It can be an amusing challenge for those trying to pronounce it, and many find it to be a fun game.

Tongue twisters have been used for centuries to challenge the listener's ability to articulate words quickly and accurately. The earliest known tongue twister was written in 1820, and since then they have become a popular game around the world.

Tongue twisters are great for practicing pronunciation or for having some fun. They can be used to help with foreign language pronunciation or to improve your accent in your native language. It is also a great exercise for improving diction and articulation.

Tongue twisters can be used as a fun way to bond with friends and family. They can be used to entertain children, or to have a laugh with your friends.

Benefits of Using Tongue Twisters

1. Tongue twisters help to improve pronunciation and enunciation.

2. They can help with speech fluency, allowing the speaker to better articulate their words.

3. Practicing tongue twisters can help to improve the speed and clarity of speech.

4. They can help to strengthen the muscles of the mouth and tongue, thus improving vocal projection.

5. Tongue twisters can also be used to help young children learn the sounds of letters and words.

How To Use Tongue Twisters for Effective Results

1. Start by selecting a tongue twister that is appropriate for your age level and skill level. If you are a beginner, try an easier tongue twister. If you are an advanced speaker, try a more difficult one.

2. Read the tongue twister slowly and out loud several times to get familiar with its rhythm and flow.

3. Once you feel comfortable with the tongue twister, practice speaking it faster. Focus on the sounds of each word and syllable and try to enunciate them clearly.

4. Record yourself speaking the tongue twister and then listen back to it. This will help you identify any areas where you may be mispronouncing words or where you can improve your speed and flow.

5. Once you feel comfortable speaking the tongue twister, practice it with friends or family. This will help you practice speaking it in a more natural way and with more confidence.

6. Finally, practice the tongue twister regularly to maintain your fluency. Try speaking it in different settings and in different voices or accents to keep it interesting.

The rest of this book will list a number of tongue twisters that you can practice with. Remember to say each one out loud, repeating each one as many times as you can and increase the speed so that you end up saying it as fast as you can.

But most of all, have fun with it and enjoy them every day. You will find that you will improve with regular practice.

List of Tongue Twisters

Q: Why did the linguist refuse to do tongue twisters?
A: Because they knew it was knot easy to say unique New York quickly and correctly!

1. A big bug bit a big black bear.
2. A big black bug bit a big black bear.
3. A big black bug bit a big black bear made the big black bear bleed blood .
4. A big bug bit the little beetle but the little beetle bit the big bug back.
5. A box of mixed biscuits.
6. A box of mixed biscuits mixed biscuits in a box.
7. A flea and a fly flew up in a flue.
8. A flea and a fly in a flue.
9. A flea and fly flew into a flue.
10. A flea and fly fought furiously.
11. A good cook could cook as much cookies as a good cook who could cook cookies.
12. A grain of sand grins grandly in the hand.
13. A noisy noise annoys an oyster.
14. A noise annoys an oyster more than a noisy noise.
15. A noise annoys an oyster but a noisy noise annoys an oyster more.
16. A noisy noise annoys an oyster but a noisy noise annoys an oyster most.
17. A noisy noise annoys the oyster but a noisy noise is what the oyster enjoys.
18. A peck of pickled peppers Peter Piper picked.
19. A proper copper coffee pot.
20. A proper cup of coffee from a proper copper coffee pot.

21. A skunk sat on a stump and thumped the stump.
22. A skunk sat on a stump and thunk the stump stunk.
23. A skunk sat on a stump the stump thought the skunk stunk.
24. A skunk spilt a skunk's milk.
25. A tree toad loved a she-toad who lived up in a tree.
26. A tutor who tooted the flute tried to tutor two tooters to toot.
27. Alliteration's amazing alliteration's amusing.
28. Betty Botter bought some butter but the butter was so bitter she bought some better butter.
29. Betty bought a bit of bitter butter but the bitter butter Betty bought was too bitter for her.
30. Betty bought some butter but the butter was so bitter.
31. Black bug's blood.
32. Can you can a can as a canner can can a can?
33. Frederico fed the radio a potato.
34. Freshly fried fly fritters frying in a fryer.
35. Fuzzy Wuzzy was a bear Fuzzy Wuzzy had no hair.
36. Fuzzy Wuzzy was a bear Fuzzy Wuzzy had no hair Fuzzy Wuzzy wasn't very fuzzy was he?
37. Greek grapes Greek grape pickers.
38. How can a clam cram in a clean cream can?
39. How can a clover cover four clovers?

40. How many cans can a cannibal nibble if a cannibal can nibble cans?
41. How many yaks could a yak pack pack if a yak pack could pack yaks?
42. How much dew does a dewdrop drop?
43. How much dew does a dewdrop drop when a dewdrop drops from the dewy dew?
44. How much dew would a dewdrop drop if a dewdrop could drop dew?
45. How much ground would a groundhog grind if a groundhog could grind ground?
46. How much oil boil can a gumboil boil if a gumboil can boil oil?
47. How much pot could a pot roast roast if a pot roast could roast pot?
48. How much wood could a woodchuck chuck if a woodchuck could chuck wood?
49. I saw Susie sitting in a shoe shine shop.
50. I saw Susie sitting in a shoeshine shop where she shines she sits and where she sits she shines.
51. I saw a kitten eating chicken in the kitchen.
52. I scream you scream we all scream for ice cream.
53. I thought a thought but the thought I thought wasn't the thought I thought I thought.
54. I wish to wash my Irish wristwatch.
55. I wish to wish the wish you wish to wish but if you wish the wish the witch wishes I won't wish the wish you wish to wish.

56. I'm not the pheasant plucker I'm the pheasant plucker's mate.
57. If Pickford's packers packed a packet of crisps would the packet of crisps that Pickford's packers packed survive for two and a half years?
58. If Stu chews shoes should Stu choose the shoes he chews?
59. If a Hottentot taught a Hottentot tot would the Hottentot tot be taught?
60. If a Hottentot taught a Hottentot tot to talk ere the tot could totter ought the Hottentot tot be taught to say aught or naught or what ought to be taught her?
61. If a dog chews shoes whose shoes does he choose?
62. If two witches were watching two watches which witch would watch which watch?
63. If you understand say "understand".
64. Irish wristwatch Swiss wristwatch.
65. Irish wristwatch Swiss wristwatch Swiss wristwatch Irish wristwatch.
66. Luke Luck likes lakes Luke's duck likes lakes Luke Luck licks lakes. Luke's duck licks lakes. Duck takes licks in lakes Luke Luck likes. Luke Luck takes licks in lakes duck likes.
67. One-One was a racehorse two-two was one too.
68. Peter Piper picked a peck of pickled peppers a peck of pickled peppers Peter Piper picked.

69. Peter Piper picked a peck of pickled peppers.
70. Peter Piper picked a peck of pickled peppers a peck of pickled peppers Peter Piper picked.
71. Picky people pick Peter Pan Peanut-Butter 'Tis the peanut-butter picky people pick.
72. Rarely is the rumpled rascal riled.
73. Red lorry green lorry.
74. Red lorry yellow lorry red lorry yellow lorry.
75. Round and round the rugged rock the ragged rascal ran.
76. Round the rugged rocks the ragged rascal ran.
77. Rub that scrub in the tub.
78. Rubber baby buggy bumpers roll down the road.
79. Seven sleepy sloths slide slowly down the slippery slope.
80. She sells seashells by the seashore.
81. She sells seashells on the seashore but the shells she sells are surely not store-bought.
82. She sells shells by the seashore.
83. She stood on the balcony inexplicably mimicking him hiccupping.
84. She stood on the balcony inexplicably mimicking him hicupping and amicably welcoming him home.
85. Silly Sally sells sea shells by the seashore.
86. Six sick hicks nick six slick bricks with picks and sticks.
87. Six sleek swans swam swiftly southwards.

88. Six slick sticks slick sticks in six slick sticks.
89. Six slimy snails slowly sliding southwards.
90. Six slippery snails slid slowly seaward.
91. Sounding by sound is a sound method of sounding sounds.
92. Swiss Miss with a Swiss kiss.
93. The lazy leopard licked the lollipop leisurely.
94. The seething sea ceaseth and thus the seething sea sufficeth us.
95. The sixth sick sheik's sixth sheep's sick.
96. Three free throws.
97. Three grey geese in a green field grazing Grey were the geese grazing in a green field.
98. Toy boat toy boat toy boat.
99. Twelve tiny turtles trekking to Tennessee.
100. Two toads in total.
101. Unique New York you vex a New Yorker.
102. Unique New York you've a tune to tune.
103. Unique New York you know you need unique New York.
104. Unique uncle's underwear unique uncle's underwear.

Conclusion

The use of vocal exercises, breathwork and tongue twisters can help speakers and singers of all levels improve their technique and performance. These techniques can be used to develop and strengthen the vocal muscles, improve vocal range and clarity, and build confidence. By practicing regularly, speakers and singers can gain control over their vocal production and create a better overall sound.

As speakers and singers strive to improve their skills, vocal exercises, breathwork and tongue twisters can provide valuable tools to help them succeed. Whether used for individual practice or as part of a group or vocal coach session, these techniques can help singers take their singing to the next level.

No matter what level of singing you are at, these techniques can help improve your vocal abilities and help you reach your goals. With a commitment to practice and dedication, vocal exercises, breathwork and tongue twisters can become a part of your regular vocal routine, helping you to become a better speaker, singer and performer.

Printed in Great Britain
by Amazon

43486252R00030